HONEY   NATURAL

REMEDIES

Honey's Healing Powers : Harnessing Nature's Sweet Nectar for Optimal Health and Well-being – Featuring Recipes, Herbal Remedies, Skincare Rituals, and Insights on Managing Diseases and Haircare.

Marie Winfrey

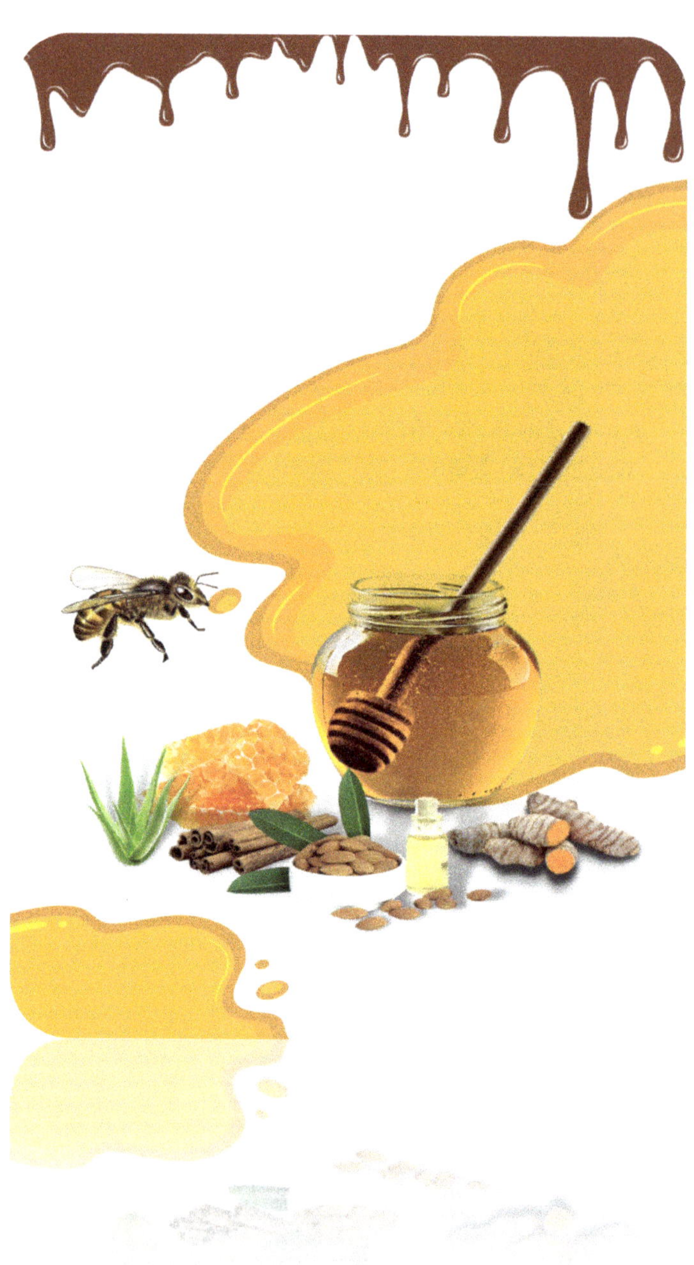

Disclaimer

The information provided in this book is based on research, personal experiences, and traditional knowledge related to honey, herbal remedies, skincare, and health management. However, individual responses to these remedies may vary, and the author and publisher do not guarantee specific outcomes.

The reader is encouraged to consult with a qualified healthcare professional before making any significant changes to their diet, lifestyle, or health practices based on the information provided in this book. The author and publisher disclaim any liability arising directly or indirectly from the use of the information contained in this book.

The information in this book is accurate and true to the best of the author's knowledge. However, the author and publisher assume no responsibility for errors, inaccuracies, or omissions. Changes may be made to the content of this book at any time without notice.

By reading this book, the reader acknowledges and agrees to the terms of this disclaimer.

Table of Contents

<u>Understanding the Power of Honey</u>

Honey has long been revered for its natural healing properties, making it a prominent player in traditional medicine and a staple in many households worldwide. The golden elixir, produced by industrious bees from the nectar of flowers, possesses a myriad of health benefits that have stood the test of time. This section delves into the rich history of honey as a natural remedy, explores the intricate composition that contributes to its healing prowess, and sheds light on the diverse types of honey and their unique benefits.

<u>The History Of Honey As A Natural Remedy</u>

The use of honey as a natural remedy can be traced back thousands of years, with its medicinal properties documented in ancient civilizations such as Egypt, Greece, and China. In these cultures, honey was not only valued for its sweet taste but revered for its therapeutic applications. Honey's antiseptic and antibacterial properties made it a crucial element in wound healing, and its consumption was believed to promote overall well-being.

In ancient Egypt, honey was used in the embalming process due to its preservative qualities. The Greek physician Hippocrates, often referred to as the father of medicine, lauded honey for its healing effects on various ailments. Throughout history, honey has been a trusted remedy for coughs, sore throats, and digestive issues. The enduring legacy of honey as a natural remedy speaks to its efficacy and the deep cultural significance attached to its use.

Composition Of Honey And Its Healing Properties

The healing properties of honey can be attributed to its intricate composition, which includes a combination of sugars, enzymes, vitamins, minerals, and antioxidants. The primary sugars in honey, fructose, and glucose, provide a natural source of energy. Enzymes such as invertase and diastase contribute to honey's digestibility, aiding in the breakdown of complex sugars.

One of the remarkable aspects of honey is its antibacterial and antifungal properties. The low water content in honey creates an inhospitable environment for microorganisms, making it a natural preservative. Additionally, honey produces hydrogen peroxide when diluted, further enhancing its antimicrobial effects. This makes honey an effective topical treatment for wounds and burns, preventing infection and promoting faster healing.

Rich in antioxidants like flavonoids and phenolic compounds, honey combats oxidative stress in the body. These antioxidants play a crucial role in reducing inflammation and protecting cells from damage. The presence of vitamins and minerals, including vitamin C, calcium, and iron, contributes to the overall nutritional profile of honey, supporting immune function and promoting general health.

Types Of Honey And Their Unique Benefits

Not all honey is created equal, as the flavor, color, and therapeutic properties can vary depending on the floral source and geographical region. Some of the most notable types of honey include Manuka, Acacia, Clover, and Buckwheat, each offering distinct benefits.

Manuka Honey

Hailing from the native Manuka bushes of New Zealand, Manuka honey is renowned for its potent antibacterial properties. It contains a compound called methylglyoxal (MGO), which sets it apart in terms of antibacterial activity. This honey is often used to treat wounds, infections, and digestive issues.

Acacia Honey

Light in color and mild in flavor, Acacia honey is derived from the nectar of the Acacia tree. Known for its high concentration of fructose, it is a preferred choice for those seeking a sweetener with a lower impact on blood sugar levels. Acacia honey is also cherished for its soothing effects on the respiratory system, making it a popular choice for alleviating coughs and throat irritation.

Clover Honey

A common variety found in many regions, Clover honey is appreciated for its versatility and mild taste. It is a rich source of antioxidants and is often used to boost overall immune function. Clover honey's antibacterial properties make it a valuable addition to wound care.

Buckwheat Honey

With its dark color and robust flavor, Buckwheat honey stands out for its high concentration of antioxidants. It is particularly effective in reducing cough symptoms and promoting better sleep. Buckwheat honey's nutritional density makes it a go-to choice for those seeking a honey variety with enhanced health benefits.

In conclusion, honey's journey as a natural remedy spans millennia, with its roots deeply embedded in the annals of traditional medicine. The intricate composition of honey, coupled with its rich history and diverse types, underscores its multifaceted role in promoting health and wellness. From wound healing to immune support, honey continues to be a timeless elixir that transcends cultural and geographical boundaries, standing as a testament to nature's remedies for the betterment of human health.

Is Honey Healthy For You?

The question of whether honey is healthy for you is one that has intrigued health enthusiasts and researchers alike. Beyond its delectable sweetness, honey's health benefits are extensive and well-documented. The natural sugars present in honey, predominantly glucose and fructose, provide a quick energy boost, making it an ideal natural sweetener for those seeking alternatives to refined sugars.

One of honey's standout qualities is its potential to support the immune system. The presence of antioxidants, such as flavonoids and polyphenols, contributes to its immune-boosting properties. These antioxidants help combat free radicals, reducing oxidative stress and inflammation in the body. As a result, regular consumption of honey may play a role in fortifying the immune response and promoting overall health.

The antimicrobial properties of honey further enhance its health-promoting characteristics. Studies have shown that honey exhibits inhibitory effects against various bacteria and fungi, showcasing its potential as a natural antibacterial agent. This has implications not only for internal health but also for the topical application of honey in wound healing and skincare.

Beyond its direct physiological effects, honey's impact on metabolic health is a subject of interest. Some research suggests that honey may have a positive influence on blood sugar levels, making it a potentially suitable option for individuals with diabetes when used in moderation. The nuanced interplay of honey's sugars and its low glycemic index contribute to its favorable profile in comparison to refined sugars.

While honey undeniably offers an array of health benefits, moderation is key. Like any natural sweetener, excessive consumption can contribute to caloric intake and potentially negate some of its positive effects. Additionally, not all honey is created equal; the quality and source of honey can influence its nutritional content. Raw, unprocessed honey retains more of its beneficial compounds compared to commercially processed varieties.

In conclusion, the question of whether honey is healthy for you can be unequivocally answered in the affirmative. Its nutritional richness, coupled with immune-boosting, antimicrobial, and potential metabolic benefits, positions honey as a valuable addition to a balanced and health-conscious diet.

Remedies For Skin

Skin Breakouts

Skin breakouts can be a challenging and often distressing issue for many individuals. The quest for effective remedies has led to exploring natural alternatives, and honey stands out as a promising solution. Its antibacterial and anti-inflammatory properties make it an excellent option for easing breakouts.

Honey's ability to reduce inflammation and bacteria on the skin contributes to its efficacy in treating breakouts. When using honey as a remedy, it is essential to choose raw, unprocessed honey for maximum benefits.

Tips

To apply, gently cleanse the affected area and then apply a thin layer of honey. Leave it on for about 15-20 minutes before rinsing off with warm water. Regular use can help soothe irritated skin, reduce redness, and promote healing.

In addition to its topical application, incorporating honey into your diet may also contribute to overall skin health. Its antioxidant properties can help combat free radicals, supporting the body's natural defenses against skin issues. Remember that individual skin types may react differently, so it's advisable to perform a patch test before widespread use.

<u>Honey And Aloe Vera Soothing Gel:</u>

For those seeking a soothing and hydrating solution, a combination of honey and aloe vera proves to be a game-changer.

- Blend together three tablespoons of aloe vera gel and one tablespoon of raw honey. This concoction becomes a calming gel that can be applied to sunburned or irritated skin.

The anti-inflammatory properties of aloe vera, combined with honey's ability to promote healing, create a potent remedy for soothing and rejuvenating the skin.

- Apply the gel generously and leave it on for 20-30 minutes before rinsing it off with cool water.

Honey And Yogurt Brightening Mask:

Achieving radiant and glowing skin is made easier with a honey and yogurt mask. In a bowl, mix two tablespoons of yogurt with one tablespoon of honey. Yogurt contains lactic acid, which gently exfoliates the skin, while honey adds a natural glow. Apply the masks lightly in your face and neck, permitting it to take a seat down for 15-20 minutes. Rinse off with lukewarm water, and pat your pores and skin dry. This remedy not only brightens the complexion but also nourishes the skin, making it an excellent addition to your beauty routine.

Honey And Oatmeal Exfoliating Scrub:

Exfoliation is a crucial step in any skincare routine, and a honey and oatmeal scrub offers a natural and gentle solution.

- Mix together two tablespoons of finely ground oatmeal with one tablespoon of honey.
- Add a small quantity of water to create a paste.
- Gently rubdown the scrub onto damp pores and skin in round motions, that specialize in regions with difficult or dry patches.

The oatmeal provides gentle exfoliation, while honey moisturizes and promotes skin renewal.

- Rinse thoroughly with warm water to reveal smoother, rejuvenated skin.

<u>Honey And Lemon Detoxifying Mask:</u>

For a detoxifying and clarifying effect, a honey and lemon mask proves to be highly effective.

- Combine one tablespoon of honey with one teaspoon of freshly squeezed lemon juice. Lemon acts as a natural astringent, helping to clarify the skin, while honey adds moisture and prevents over-drying.

- Apply the mixture to your face, avoiding the eye area, and leave it on for 10-15 minutes.
- Rinse off with lukewarm water and pat your face dry.

This mask is ideal for those looking to address issues such as excess oiliness and occasional breakouts.

<u>Honey and Yogurt Face Mask for Acne</u>

Acne is a common skin condition that can affect individuals of all ages. Honey, known for its antibacterial and anti-inflammatory properties, can be combined with yogurt to create a nourishing face mask that may help combat acne. In this section, we will provide detailed directions for creating and using a honey and yogurt face mask as part of a holistic approach to skincare.

<u>Ingredients And Preparation:</u>

Gather two tablespoons of raw honey and two tablespoons of plain, unsweetened yogurt. Raw honey is preferred for its unprocessed nature, while yogurt contains lactic acid, which can aid in exfoliation. Mix the honey and yogurt thoroughly in a bowl until a smooth and consistent paste is formed.

<u>Cleansing the Face:</u>

Before applying the mask, ensure your face is clean and free from makeup or impurities. Use a gentle cleanser appropriate for your skin type to prepare the skin for the mask. Pat your face dry with a clean towel.

<u>Application of the Mask:</u>

Using clean fingers or a brush, apply the honey and yogurt mixture evenly to your face, avoiding the eye and mouth areas. The mask should be applied in a thick, even layer to maximize its effectiveness. Take care to cover any areas prone to acne breakouts.

<u>Relaxation Period:</u>

Allow the mask to sit on your face for 15-20 minutes. This time allows the honey and yogurt to penetrate the skin, delivering their beneficial properties. While the mask is on, take the opportunity to relax and unwind.

<u>Rinsing Off the Mask:</u>

After the recommended duration, gently rinse the mask off with lukewarm water. Use circular motions to massage the mask into your skin as you rinse, promoting further exfoliation. Pat your face dry with a clean towel.

<u>Moisturizing:</u>

Follow up the mask treatment with a suitable moisturizer to lock in hydration. Consider using a non-comedogenic moisturizer to prevent clogging pores. This step is essential for maintaining skin balance after the mask application.

<u>Frequency of Use:</u>

The honey and yogurt face mask can be applied 1-2 times a week, depending on individual skin sensitivity and response. Consistent use over time may help reduce acne inflammation, minimize breakouts, and improve overall skin texture.

<u>Cautionary Notes:</u>

Conduct a patch test before applying the mask to your entire face, especially if you have sensitive skin. If irritation occurs, discontinue use. Additionally, it is advisable to consult with a dermatologist if you have severe or persistent acne concerns.

The honey and yogurt face mask offers a natural and gentle approach to managing acne, harnessing the combined benefits of honey's antimicrobial properties and yogurt's exfoliating effects. When incorporated into a regular skincare routine and complemented by good hygiene practices, this mask can contribute to clearer, healthier-looking skin over time.

Insect Bite Relief

Insect bites can cause discomfort, itching, and sometimes allergic reactions. Finding a natural remedy for insect bite relief is essential, and honey's anti-inflammatory and soothing properties make it an excellent candidate.

<u>Tips</u>

To alleviate the discomfort associated with insect bites, apply a small amount of raw honey directly to the affected area. The anti-inflammatory properties help reduce swelling, while the sticky texture creates a protective barrier, preventing further irritation. Honey's natural antiseptic qualities can also aid in preventing infection, promoting faster healing.

For a more cooling sensation, consider mixing honey with aloe vera gel before applying. Aloe vera complements honey's soothing properties and enhances the overall relief. This combination can be particularly effective for mosquito bites, bee stings, or other common insect-related irritations.

As with any remedy, individual reactions may vary, so it's advisable to monitor for allergic responses. If the symptoms persist or worsen, seeking professional medical advice is recommended.

Cinnamon Honey: For Overall Wellness

The combination of cinnamon and honey has been revered for its potential health benefits for centuries. This dynamic duo is known for its antioxidant, anti-inflammatory, and antimicrobial properties, making it a popular choice for promoting overall wellness.

Cinnamon honey is not only a delicious addition to your culinary repertoire but also a powerful health tonic. The antioxidants in cinnamon help combat oxidative stress, while honey's antimicrobial properties contribute to a strengthened immune system. This combination is believed to have potential cardiovascular benefits by positively impacting cholesterol levels and blood pressure.

To incorporate cinnamon honey into your daily routine, consider adding a teaspoon of this mixture to your morning tea or drizzling it over yogurt. It's important to note that while cinnamon is generally safe in moderation, excessive consumption may lead to health issues. As with any natural remedy, it's advisable to consult with a healthcare professional, especially if you have pre-existing health conditions or are taking medications.

Ginger Honey: For Sore Stomach

A sore stomach can disrupt daily activities and affect overall well-being. Ginger honey emerges as a natural remedy with anti-inflammatory and digestive properties that can help alleviate stomach discomfort.

Tips

To prepare ginger honey for a sore stomach, start by peeling and grating fresh ginger. Mix the grated ginger with an equal amount of honey, creating a potent combination of anti-inflammatory gingerols and soothing honey. The recommended dosage is one to two teaspoons of this mixture, taken as needed. It can be ingested directly or added to warm water to make a soothing ginger honey tea.

Ginger works by reducing inflammation in the stomach lining, easing nausea, and promoting overall digestive health. Honey complements this by providing a coating effect on the irritated stomach lining, further reducing discomfort. This natural remedy is particularly beneficial for soothing symptoms of indigestion, bloating, and mild stomach upset.

It's important to note that while ginger and honey are generally considered safe, individual responses may vary. Pregnant individuals, those with pre-existing medical conditions, or those taking medications should consult with a healthcare professional before incorporating this remedy into their routine.

Clove Honey For Toothache

Toothaches can be excruciating, and seeking natural remedies for relief is a common approach. Clove honey, a combination of honey and clove oil, offers a potential solution due to its analgesic and anti-inflammatory properties.

<u>Tips</u>

To create clove honey for toothache relief, mix a few drops of clove oil with a teaspoon of honey. Clove oil contains eugenol, a natural compound known for its pain-relieving and antibacterial properties. The honey serves as a carrier for the clove oil, enhancing its application and providing additional soothing effects.

<u>Application</u>

Apply the clove honey mixture directly to the affected tooth and surrounding gums. Gently massage the area for a few minutes, allowing the remedy to penetrate and provide relief. The antimicrobial properties of both honey and clove oil contribute to preventing potential infections and promoting oral health.

While this natural remedy can offer temporary relief, it is essential to address the underlying cause of the toothache. Consultation with a dentist is crucial for a comprehensive evaluation and appropriate treatment. Additionally, individuals with allergies or sensitivities should perform a patch test before applying the mixture extensively.

Apple Cider Vinegar And Honey For Acid Reflux

In the pursuit of natural remedies for health and wellness, the combination of apple cider vinegar and honey has emerged as a potent solution for managing acid reflux. Acid reflux, characterized by a burning sensation in the chest caused by stomach acid flowing back into the esophagus, is a common ailment affecting millions worldwide. This dynamic duo, consisting of the acidity-balancing properties of apple cider vinegar and the soothing nature of honey, provides a holistic approach to alleviating acid reflux symptoms.

Apple Cider Vinegar (ACV):

Apple cider vinegar is renowned for its myriad health benefits, and its effectiveness in addressing acid reflux is no exception. The acidity of ACV helps balance the pH levels in the stomach, preventing the excessive production of acid that leads to reflux. Additionally, ACV promotes digestive health by encouraging the production of digestive enzymes, facilitating smoother digestion and reducing the likelihood of reflux.

<u>Honey:</u>

The inclusion of honey in this remedy serves a dual purpose. First and foremost, honey is known for its natural anti-inflammatory properties. It soothes the irritated lining of the esophagus, providing relief from the discomfort associated with acid reflux. Secondly, honey acts as a natural sweetener, making the remedy more palatable and easier to incorporate into one's daily routine.

<u>Direction For Use With Dosage:</u>

For optimal results, it is recommended to mix one to two tablespoons of raw, unfiltered apple cider vinegar with an equal amount of honey in a glass of warm water. This concoction should be consumed 15-30 minutes before meals to preemptively address acid reflux. The warm water aids in the soothing delivery of the remedy to the digestive system.

It is crucial to use raw, unfiltered apple cider vinegar containing the "mother," a colony of beneficial bacteria, enzymes, and proteins. This ensures that the vinegar retains its full spectrum of health-promoting properties.

For those new to this remedy, starting with a lower dosage and gradually increasing it as tolerance develops is advisable. Persons with pre-existing health conditions or on medication should consult a healthcare professional before incorporating this remedy into their routine.

Consistency is key when using apple cider vinegar and honey for acid reflux. Integrating this natural remedy into a daily routine can contribute to long-term relief from acid reflux symptoms. However, it is essential to complement this remedy with a balanced diet, proper hydration, and other lifestyle adjustments for comprehensive management of acid reflux.

the combination of apple cider vinegar and honey stands as a promising natural remedy for acid reflux, offering a holistic and sustainable approach to managing this common ailment. As with any health regimen, consultation with a healthcare professional is advised, especially for those with underlying health conditions.

Honey Heel Moisturizer For Dry, Cracked Heels

Dry, cracked heels can be both painful and unsightly, often stemming from factors such as dehydration, lack of proper foot care, or certain medical conditions. The Honey Heel Moisturizer, a natural remedy harnessing the healing properties of honey, emerges as a nurturing solution to combat this common foot ailment.

Nature's Gift: Honey's Healing Properties

Honey, a golden elixir produced by bees from the nectar of flowers, has been revered for its medicinal properties for centuries. Its natural antibacterial and antifungal qualities make it an ideal ingredient for healing and rejuvenating the skin. When applied to dry, cracked heels, honey works to moisturize, soften, and promote the healing of damaged skin.

Tips:

Creating a Honey Heel Moisturizer at home is a simple yet effective process. Begin by mixing equal parts of raw honey and a nourishing carrier oil, such as coconut or olive oil. The combination of honey's humectant properties and the emollient nature of the carrier oil creates a powerful moisturizing blend.

Application:

Before applying the moisturizer, it is essential to cleanse the feet thoroughly to remove any dirt or impurities. Soaking the feet in warm water for a few minutes can help soften the skin, making it more receptive to the moisturizing treatment.

Once the feet are clean and dry, generously apply the Honey Heel Moisturizer to the affected areas, paying special attention to the heels. Gently massage the mixture into the skin, allowing the healing properties of honey to penetrate deeply.

For enhanced results, consider covering the moisturized feet with clean socks and leaving the mixture on overnight. This not only prevents the moisturizer from transferring onto surfaces but also allows for prolonged absorption and healing.

<u>Incorporating into Daily Foot Care Routine:</u>

Consistency is key when treating dry, cracked heels. Incorporating the Honey Heel Moisturizer into a daily foot care routine can prevent the recurrence of dryness and maintain soft, supple skin. Regular application, especially after showering or bathing, helps lock in moisture and supports the skin's natural healing processes.

Additionally, staying hydrated, wearing comfortable and breathable footwear, and exfoliating the feet periodically can complement the effects of the Honey Heel Moisturizer. Individuals with diabetes or other medical conditions affecting foot health should consult a healthcare professional before adopting new foot care practices.

the Honey Heel Moisturizer stands as a testament to nature's ability to provide effective solutions for common ailments. Harnessing the healing properties of honey, this remedy offers a natural and nurturing approach to combat dry, cracked heels, promoting not only skin health but overall well-being.

Honey For Sore Throat

Sore throats are a common ailment that can be both uncomfortable and disruptive to daily life. Honey, a natural sweetener with potent medicinal properties, has been recognized for centuries as a soothing remedy for sore throats. In this section, we will explore the proper directions for using honey to alleviate sore throat symptoms, along with recommended dosage guidelines.

Tips

Selecting the Right Honey:

To maximize the therapeutic benefits, it is crucial to choose high-quality, raw honey. Raw honey contains various enzymes, antioxidants, and antimicrobial compounds that contribute to its healing properties. Look for locally sourced honey when possible, as it may offer additional benefits due to exposure to local allergens.

Dosage Guidelines:

The recommended dosage of honey for sore throat relief can vary based on age and individual preferences. For adults, a common approach is to consume one to two tablespoons of honey every few hours, either directly or by adding it to warm water or herbal tea. For children aged one year and older, a teaspoon of honey can be given as needed. It's important to note that honey should not be given to infants under one year of age due to the risk of infant botulism.

Direct Consumption:

For immediate relief, individuals can consume honey directly from the spoon or mix it with warm water or tea. The warmth of the liquid helps soothe the throat, while the honey's antimicrobial properties may aid in combating infection. Slowly sipping the mixture allows the honey to coat the throat, providing a protective and calming effect.

Honey and Lemon Combination:

Combining honey with freshly squeezed lemon juice enhances its effectiveness in relieving sore throats. Lemon adds vitamin C and acidity, which can help break down mucus and provide additional relief. Mix one tablespoon of honey with the juice of half a lemon in a cup of warm water for a soothing drink.

Gargling With Honey:

Gargling with a honey solution can be beneficial for targeting the back of the throat. Mix one tablespoon of honey with warm water and a pinch of salt. Gargle the solution for 15-30 seconds, ensuring it reaches the affected areas. Repeat this process several times a day for optimal results.

Incorporating Honey Into Herbal Teas:

Herbal teas, such as chamomile or peppermint, combined with honey, can provide dual benefits.

These teas have their own therapeutic properties, while honey complements their effects. Brew a cup of herbal tea and add honey to taste for a comforting and healing beverage.

Honey's Role in Hair Care

In the pursuit of vibrant and healthy hair, the integration of natural remedies has gained significant popularity. Among these remedies, honey stands out as a versatile and potent ingredient for promoting lustrous locks. This part explores the manifold benefits of honey in hair care, delving into the art of creating honey infusions for shiny and healthy hair, as well as addressing common scalp issues through the application of honey-based hair masks.

Honey Infusions For Shiny And Healthy Hair:

Honey, a natural humectant, possesses inherent moisturizing properties that can transform dull and lifeless hair into a radiant mane. The creation of honey infusions offers a simple yet effective approach to harnessing its benefits for hair health.

<u>Begin with Quality Ingredients:</u>

To embark on the journey of honey-infused hair care, it is crucial to start with high-quality honey. Opt for raw, unprocessed honey, as it retains its natural enzymes and nutrients that contribute to hair vitality. Additionally, consider incorporating complementary ingredients such as coconut oil, aloe vera, or essential oils to enhance the infusion's efficacy.

<u>The Art of Infusion:</u>

Creating a honey infusion involves blending the chosen ingredients in a harmonious combination. Begin by heating a measured amount of honey gently, ensuring it retains its raw properties. Mix it with the selected oils or extracts, paying attention to consistency. The goal is to form a smooth and homogeneous mixture that is easy to apply to the hair.

Application Techniques:

Applying honey infusions to the hair requires a strategic approach. Start by dampening the hair slightly, allowing for better absorption of the infusion. Section the hair and apply the mixture evenly, ensuring that each strand receives the nourishing benefits. Leave the infusion on for at least 30 minutes to allow the hair to absorb the nutrients fully.

Rinse and Revel:

After the designated period, rinse the hair thoroughly with lukewarm water. Shampoo and condition as usual to remove any residue. The result is hair that not only looks lustrous but also feels soft and revitalized. Regular application of honey infusions can contribute to long-term hair health and shine.

Treating Scalp Issues With Honey-Based Hair Masks

Beyond imparting shine, honey proves to be a powerful ally in addressing common scalp issues. The use of honey-based hair masks offers a holistic solution to problems such as dandruff, dry scalp, and irritation.

<u>Nourishing the Scalp:</u>

Honey's natural antibacterial and antifungal properties make it an excellent choice for combatting scalp issues. When crafting honey-based hair masks, consider combining honey with ingredients like yogurt, apple cider vinegar, or tea tree oil. These additions not only enhance the mask's effectiveness but also contribute to a healthier scalp environment.

Banishing Dandruff with Honey:

Dandruff, a persistent concern for many, can be alleviated through the application of a honey-based mask. Formulate a mixture of honey, a few drops of tea tree oil, and yogurt. Tea tree oil's antifungal properties work synergistically with honey to eliminate dandruff-causing agents. Massage the mask into the scalp and leave it on for 45 minutes before rinsing thoroughly.

<u>Hydration for Dry Scalp:</u>

Dry scalp often leads to itching and irritation. A honey and aloe vera mask can provide much-needed hydration. Aloe vera's soothing properties, combined with honey's moisturizing effects, create a potent remedy for dry scalp. Apply the mask, massage gently, and let it sit for 30 minutes before rinsing. Regular use can restore moisture balance and alleviate dryness.

<u>Soothing Irritated Scalp:</u>

For those with sensitive or irritated scalps, a honey and chamomile mask can offer relief. Chamomile's anti-inflammatory properties complement honey's soothing effects. Mix honey with chamomile tea and apply the mask to the scalp. Leave it on for 20-30 minutes, allowing the calming blend to work its magic.

<u>Consistency is Key:</u>

Achieving lasting results requires consistency in application. Incorporate honey-based hair masks into your hair care routine on a weekly basis, adjusting the frequency based on your scalp's needs. With time, the masks can contribute to a healthier scalp and stronger, more resilient hair.

In the realm of natural remedies for hair care, honey emerges as a versatile and effective solution. From infusions that enhance shine to masks that address various scalp issues, honey's benefits extend beyond its delectable taste. By incorporating these practices into your routine, you can unlock the full potential of honey for achieving and maintaining lustrous locks and a healthy scalp.

Honey And Turmeric For Joint Pain

The Science Behind Honey And Turmeric:

Both honey and turmeric have been recognized for their anti-inflammatory and antioxidant properties. Honey, a natural sweetener produced by bees, contains compounds that exhibit anti-inflammatory effects, helping to reduce swelling and discomfort in joints. Turmeric, on the other hand, is renowned for curcumin, its active ingredient with potent anti-inflammatory and antioxidant properties. Scientific studies have suggested that the combination of honey and turmeric may offer a synergistic effect, enhancing their individual benefits and making them a formidable duo for combating joint pain.

Tips For Choosing The Right Honey And Turmeric:

Before delving into the practical aspects of using honey and turmeric for joint pain relief, it's essential to choose high-quality ingredients. When selecting honey, opt for raw, unprocessed varieties, as they retain more of the beneficial compounds. Manuka honey, derived from the nectar of the Manuka tree, is particularly praised for its potent anti-inflammatory and antibacterial properties.

Similarly, when choosing turmeric, look for high-quality organic turmeric powder or fresh turmeric root. The active compound, curcumin, is more concentrated in turmeric powder, making it a convenient option for incorporating into various recipes.

<u>Consuming Honey And Turmeric:</u>

There are several ways to incorporate honey and turmeric into your daily routine to harness their joint pain-relieving benefits:

<u>Golden Honey Paste:</u>

Mix one tablespoon of turmeric powder with a quarter cup of raw honey to form a paste.

Consume a teaspoon of this golden honey paste daily, preferably in the morning.

Gradually increase the dosage if needed, under the guidance of a healthcare professional.

<u>Turmeric Tea with Honey:</u>

Brew a cup of turmeric tea using turmeric powder or grated fresh turmeric.

Add a teaspoon of honey for sweetness and enhanced therapeutic effects.

Enjoy this soothing tea regularly, especially during periods of increased joint discomfort.

Turmeric and Honey Smoothie:

Blend fresh turmeric root or turmeric powder with fruits, yogurt, and a tablespoon of honey.

Incorporate this smoothie into your breakfast routine for a delicious and nutritious start to your day.

Honey And Turmeric Infused Water:

Mix a teaspoon of turmeric powder and honey in a glass of warm water.

Stir well and consume this concoction on an empty stomach for potential joint pain relief.

Precautions And Considerations:

While honey and turmeric are generally considered safe, it's crucial to exercise caution and consult with a healthcare professional before incorporating them into your routine, especially if you have existing health conditions or are taking medications. Turmeric may interact with certain medications, and excessive consumption can lead to digestive issues.

Additionally, persons allergic to bee products should avoid honey. Pregnant or breastfeeding women should seek medical advice before using these remedies.

Anti-Inflammatory Wonders Of Honey And Turmeric

At the heart of this remedy lies the marriage of two extraordinary natural ingredients – honey and turmeric. Both have been revered across cultures for their medicinal properties, and when combined, they create a potent concoction with anti-inflammatory superpowers. Honey, known for its antimicrobial and anti-inflammatory properties, acts as a soothing agent, while turmeric, with its active compound curcumin, adds an extra layer of anti-inflammatory prowess.

Turmeric, often referred to as "Indian saffron," has been used in traditional medicine for centuries. Its vibrant yellow hue is attributed to curcumin, a bioactive compound with proven anti-inflammatory and antioxidant effects. When paired with honey, these ingredients form a formidable alliance that not only tantalizes the taste buds but also addresses the root causes of inflammation in the body.

<u>Crafting Honey And Turmeric Éclairs:</u>

Creating the perfect Honey and Turmeric Éclairs requires a delicate balance of flavors and a meticulous approach to harnessing the full potential of these natural remedies. Here's a step-by-step guide to crafting these delectable treats for maximum anti-inflammatory benefits:

<u>Ingredients:</u>

- Pâte à Choux (Choux pastry)
- Honey and Turmeric Cream Filling
- Honey Glaze

<u>Directions:</u>

<u>Pâte à Choux:</u>

Begin by preparing the choux pastry. Combine water, butter, salt, and a touch of honey in a saucepan. Once it reaches a boil, add flour and stir vigorously until a smooth dough forms. Allow it to cool slightly before incorporating eggs, one at a time. Pipe the dough onto a baking sheet and bake until golden brown.

<u>Honey and Turmeric Cream Filling:</u>

In a mixing bowl, whip together heavy cream, honey, and a generous amount of turmeric. The goal is to achieve a velvety, golden-hued cream with a subtle sweetness. Adjust the turmeric to your liking, keeping in mind both flavor and the desired anti-inflammatory effect.

<u>Assembly:</u>

Once the choux pastry has cooled, cut it in half horizontally. Fill a piping bag with the Honey and Turmeric Cream Filling and generously pipe it onto the bottom halves of the éclairs. Gently place the other halves on top, creating a sandwich. Drizzle the assembled éclairs with a honey glaze for an extra touch of sweetness and anti-inflammatory goodness.

Tips For Consumption:

Consistency is Key: Incorporate these éclairs into your routine consistently for the best results. The anti-inflammatory properties of honey and turmeric compound over time.

Mindful Consumption:

Enjoy these treats mindfully, savoring each bite. The joy of indulging in a delicious dessert can complement the therapeutic effects of the honey and turmeric.

Pair With Tea:

Consider pairing your Honey and Turmeric Éclairs with a soothing cup of herbal tea. Certain teas, such as chamomile or ginger, can further enhance the anti-inflammatory benefits of this delightful treat.

<u>Balance With A Healthy Lifestyle:</u>

While these éclairs offer a natural remedy for inflammation, it's essential to maintain a well-rounded, healthy lifestyle. Incorporate a nutrient-rich diet, regular exercise, and sufficient sleep for holistic well-being.

Lavender Honey For Stress Reduction

Understanding Lavender Honey:

Lavender honey is a distinct variety known for its unique flavor profile, which is a harmonious blend of the sweetness of honey and the floral, earthy notes of lavender. The process of collecting this honey involves bees foraging on lavender plants, imparting the honey with the plant's natural compounds. These compounds, including linalool and linalyl acetate, contribute to lavender honey's calming properties, making it an ideal choice for stress reduction.

<u>**Tips For Choosing Quality Lavender Honey:**</u>

Selecting high-quality lavender honey is crucial to maximize its stress-relieving benefits. When purchasing, opt for organic and raw varieties to ensure that the honey retains its natural enzymes and therapeutic properties. Look for honey sourced from reputable beekeepers or local farmers who prioritize sustainable and ethical beekeeping practices.

<u>Incorporating Lavender Honey Into Your Routine For Stress Reduction</u>

<u>Tea Infusion:</u>

One of the simplest and most soothing ways to enjoy lavender honey is by adding it to your favorite tea. Choose calming herbal teas like chamomile or lavender tea itself for a double dose of relaxation. Stir in a teaspoon of lavender honey, allowing it to dissolve and infuse its flavor into the warm beverage. Sipping on this aromatic tea can create a serene ritual that promotes mental tranquility.

Spread on Toast or Crackers:

Lavender honey can be spread on whole-grain toast or crackers as a delightful and nutritious snack. The subtle floral notes complement the nuttiness of the grains, creating a balanced and satisfying treat. This option is not only a delicious way to incorporate lavender honey into your diet but also provides a quick and convenient stress-relieving option for busy days.

Yogurt Parfait with Lavender Honey:

Elevate your yogurt parfait by drizzling lavender honey over the layers of yogurt, granola, and fresh fruits. This not only enhances the flavor but also adds a therapeutic dimension to your breakfast or snack. Yogurt provides probiotics for gut health, while lavender honey contributes its stress-reducing properties, making this a wholesome and nourishing option.

<u>DIY Lavender Honey Elixir:</u>

Create a custom lavender honey elixir by combining warm water, a tablespoon of lavender honey, and a squeeze of fresh lemon juice. Stir well to dissolve the honey and enjoy this soothing concoction. The combination of honey's natural sweetness, lavender's calming essence, and the invigorating citrus notes of lemon makes for a refreshing and stress-relieving drink.

<u>Lavender Honey and Nut Butter Pairing:</u>

Combine the richness of nut butter with the sweetness of lavender honey for a delightful pairing. Spread almond or cashew butter on whole-grain bread and drizzle lavender honey on top. This wholesome combination provides a balanced blend of protein, healthy fats, and the calming properties of lavender honey, making it a satiating snack that can also help alleviate stress.

<u>**Precautions and Considerations:**</u>

While lavender honey offers numerous benefits for stress reduction, it's essential to exercise caution, especially for individuals with allergies to bee products. Consult with a healthcare professional if you have any concerns or pre-existing medical conditions. Additionally, moderation is key, as excessive consumption of honey can contribute to an increase in calorie intake.

Lavender honey, with its unique flavor and stress-relieving properties, serves as a valuable addition to the toolkit of natural remedies for health and wellness. By incorporating this delightful honey into various aspects of your daily routine, you can not only enjoy its therapeutic benefits but also create moments of calm and relaxation amidst the demands of modern life. Whether sipped in a cup of tea, spread on toast, or integrated into a custom elixir, lavender honey stands as a testament to nature's ability to provide both pleasure and healing.

Cinnamon And Honey Synergy For Diabetes Management

the combination of cinnamon and honey has garnered significant attention, particularly in the context of diabetes management. This dynamic duo is celebrated for its potential to help regulate blood sugar levels and improve insulin sensitivity.

Understanding The Individual Benefits

Cinnamon, derived from the inner bark of trees belonging to the Cinnamomum family, has been studied for its potential antidiabetic effects. The active compounds, such as cinnamaldehyde, may play a role in improving insulin sensitivity and reducing blood sugar levels. Moreover, cinnamon is rich in antioxidants, which can contribute to overall health by combating oxidative stress.

Honey, a natural sweetener produced by bees, is not only a source of energy but also boasts various health-promoting properties. Studies suggest that honey may have antidiabetic effects, potentially helping to lower blood sugar levels. Additionally, honey exhibits anti-inflammatory and antioxidant properties, supporting the body's overall immune function.

Synergy In Diabetes Management

When cinnamon and honey are combined, their synergistic effects can create a powerful natural remedy for diabetes management. Cinnamon may enhance insulin sensitivity, allowing cells to better respond to insulin, while honey provides a natural sweetener with potential antidiabetic properties. Together, they work in harmony to address multiple aspects of diabetes, making it a holistic approach to complement conventional treatments.

Tips for Incorporating Cinnamon and Honey into Your Routine

Select Quality Ingredients:

Ensure that you choose high-quality cinnamon and honey for optimal benefits. Look for organic, pure honey and cinnamon free from additives or artificial substances.

<u>Dosage Considerations:</u>
It's crucial to consume these ingredients in moderation. Excessive intake may lead to unwanted effects. Consult with a healthcare professional to determine an appropriate dosage based on your individual health condition.

<u>Types Of Cinnamon:</u>
There are different types of cinnamon, with Ceylon and Cassia being the most common. Ceylon cinnamon is often considered the "true" cinnamon and may be a preferable choice for its lower coumarin content. However, both types have shown potential health benefits.

<u>Incorporate Into Meals:</u>

Sprinkle cinnamon on various dishes, such as oatmeal, yogurt, or smoothies. Mix honey into beverages like tea or use it as a natural sweetener in recipes. Combining them in warm water with a dash of cinnamon can make a soothing and healthful drink.

<u>Monitor Blood Sugar Levels:</u>

Regularly monitor your blood sugar levels, especially if you are using cinnamon and honey as part of your diabetes management plan. This will help you assess the effectiveness of the remedy and make any necessary adjustments.

<u>Consulting With A Healthcare Professional:</u>

Before making significant changes to your diet or incorporating new natural remedies, consult with your healthcare provider. They can provide personalized advice based on your specific health condition and ensure that the cinnamon and honey combination aligns with your overall diabetes management plan.

<u>Daily Routine</u>

To effectively harness the potential benefits of cinnamon and honey for diabetes management, consider the following daily routine:

Morning Routine:

Start your day with a warm beverage by adding a teaspoon of cinnamon and a tablespoon of honey to a cup of hot water. This can be a soothing and healthful alternative to traditional sweeteners in your morning tea or coffee.

Meal Enhancements:

Sprinkle cinnamon on your breakfast foods, such as oatmeal or whole-grain toast. Use honey as a natural sweetener in recipes, ensuring that it complements your overall dietary goals.

Afternoon Pick-Me-Up:

Incorporate a midday snack that includes the dynamic duo. Consider pairing a piece of fruit with a small drizzle of honey and a sprinkle of cinnamon for a tasty and healthful treat.

Evening Ritual:

Wind down your day with a calming cup of cinnamon and honey tea. This can be achieved by steeping a cinnamon stick in hot water and adding a teaspoon of honey. This not only aids in diabetes management but also promotes relaxation.

Consistency is Key:

Incorporate cinnamon and honey into your daily routine consistently to experience potential benefits over time. Remember that natural remedies often require time to show noticeable effects, so be patient and persistent.

Bad Breath: A Sweet Solution For Oral Odor

Bad breath, or halitosis, can be a persistent concern that affects social interactions and self-confidence. Honey, with its antibacterial properties and soothing effects, presents a natural remedy to address the root causes of bad breath while providing a sweet solution for oral hygiene.

<u>Ingredients:</u>

- 1 teaspoon of raw, Manuka honey (preferred for its potent antibacterial properties)
- Warm water
- Optional: A pinch of cinnamon powder

<u>Directions:</u>

Mix one teaspoon of raw Manuka honey into a cup of warm water.

Optionally, add a pinch of cinnamon powder to enhance the antibacterial effects.

Use this honey-water mixture as a mouthwash, swishing it around the mouth for at least 30 seconds before spitting it out.

Honey's antibacterial properties inhibit the growth of bacteria in the mouth, reducing the chances of plaque formation and gum disease, both contributors to bad breath. Manuka honey, in particular, is renowned for its potent antibacterial qualities, making it an excellent choice for addressing oral odor.

Regular use of honey as a natural mouthwash not only combats bad breath but also soothes the oral tissues, promoting overall oral health. This approach aligns with the principles of natural remedies, providing an alternative to commercial mouthwashes laden with artificial chemicals.

Honey for Cough: Nature's Golden Elixir for Respiratory Relief

When it comes to soothing a persistent cough, honey stands out as a time-honored remedy, offering a natural and delicious alternative to over-the-counter cough syrups. Honey's unique combination of antioxidants, antimicrobial properties, and soothing effects makes it an effective choice for alleviating cough symptoms.

Ingredients:

- 1 to 2 tablespoons of raw, local honey
- Optional: Freshly squeezed lemon juice
- Warm water

<u>Directions:</u>

- Measure 1 to 2 tablespoons of raw, local honey.
- Optionally, mix in a teaspoon of freshly squeezed lemon juice for added vitamin C and flavor.
- Consume the honey mixture directly or dilute it in a cup of warm water for a comforting drink.

Honey's thick consistency helps coat the throat, providing relief from irritation that triggers coughing. Its antimicrobial properties contribute to overall respiratory health by combating infections. The addition of lemon juice not only enhances the flavor but also brings its own set of antioxidants and immune-boosting benefits.

This natural cough remedy is especially valuable for individuals seeking alternatives to traditional cough syrups, which often contain artificial ingredients. Embracing honey as a go-to solution aligns with the holistic approach to health and wellness, harnessing the power of nature for respiratory comfort.

Remedy For Insomenia

the combination of honey and herbs stands out as a potent solution for addressing insomnia, a prevalent sleep disorder affecting millions worldwide. This holistic approach leverages the soothing properties of honey and the sleep-inducing qualities of carefully chosen herbs.

Understanding Insomnia:

Insomnia, characterized by difficulty falling or staying asleep, can have detrimental effects on both physical and mental well-being. Factors such as stress, lifestyle choices, and environmental influences contribute to this sleep disorder.

While pharmaceutical interventions are available, a growing number of individuals seek natural alternatives to alleviate their insomnia symptoms, and the honey with herbs remedy presents an appealing option.

<u>**Key Ingredients**</u>

Raw Honey: Raw honey, prized for its natural sweetness and numerous health benefits, serves as the base for this remedy. Packed with antioxidants and anti-inflammatory properties, raw honey helps reduce inflammation and promotes overall well-being. Its natural sugars can also contribute to the release of serotonin, a precursor to melatonin, the sleep-inducing hormone.

<u>Lavender:</u>

 Lavender, known for its calming and aromatic qualities, plays a crucial role in combating insomnia. Its essential oils contain compounds such as linalool and linalyl acetate, which have been shown to reduce anxiety and induce relaxation, promoting a restful night's sleep.

<u>Chamomile:</u>

 Chamomile, a popular herb with mild sedative effects, aids in relaxation and can alleviate symptoms of insomnia. Its properties are attributed to apigenin, an antioxidant that binds to certain receptors in the brain, promoting sleepiness and reducing insomnia symptoms.

<u>Valerian Root:</u>

Valerian root has been used for hundreds of years as a herbal treatment for sleep disorders. Its compounds, including valerenic acid, interact with gamma-aminobutyric acid (GABA) receptors in the brain, promoting a calming effect and facilitating better sleep.

Preparation And Directions

To create the honey with herbs remedy for insomnia, follow these step-by-step instructions:

<u>Ingredients:</u>

- 1 cup of raw honey
- 2 tablespoons of dried lavender
- 2 tablespoons of dried chamomile flowers
- 1 tablespoon of valerian root

Directions:

<u>Choose High-Quality Ingredients:</u>

Select organic and high-quality herbs to ensure the potency and effectiveness of the remedy.

<u>Combine Herbs and Honey:</u>

In a clean, glass jar, mix the dried lavender, chamomile flowers, and valerian root with raw honey. Stir well to ensure the herbs are evenly distributed.

<u>Infusion Process:</u>

Allow the mixture to infuse for at least two weeks in a cool, dark place. This allows the honey to absorb the beneficial properties of the herbs.

<u>Strain the Mixture:</u>

After the infusion period, strain the mixture to remove the solid herb particles. This can be done using a fine mesh strainer or cheesecloth.

<u>Storage:</u>

Transfer the strained honey-herb infusion into a clean, airtight glass jar for storage. Ensure the jar is stored away from direct sunlight.

<u>Usage Guidelines:</u>

Dosage:

Consume one tablespoon of the honey-herb mixture approximately 30 minutes before bedtime.

<u>Consistency is Key:</u>

For optimal results, incorporate this remedy into your nightly routine consistently.

The honey with herbs remedy for insomnia offers a natural and holistic approach to addressing sleep disorders. By combining the soothing properties of raw honey with the calming effects of lavender, chamomile, and valerian root, this remedy aims to promote relaxation and improve overall sleep quality.

Honey For Weight Loss: A Sweet Solution To Shedding Pounds

The natural sweetness of honey, along with its potential benefits such as improved metabolism and appetite regulation, makes it a versatile and delicious option for those looking to shed pounds. As with any weight loss strategy, consistency and balance are key, and it is advisable to consult with a healthcare professional or nutritionist before making significant changes to your diet.

Ingredients

To harness the weight-loss potential of honey, it is essential to select high-quality, raw honey. Raw honey retains its natural enzymes and antioxidants, which may be compromised during the processing of commercial honey. Additionally, for an extra boost, you can combine honey with other ingredients known for their weight loss properties, such as lemon, cinnamon, or apple cider vinegar.

Lemon and Honey Infusion:

A refreshing and effective way to consume honey for weight loss is by preparing a simple lemon and honey infusion. Mix two tablespoons of raw honey with the juice of half a lemon in a glass of lukewarm water. Stir well and consume this concoction on an empty stomach in the morning. Lemon adds vitamin C and acidity, which may enhance metabolism, while honey provides a natural sweetness and potential appetite-suppressant effects.

Cinnamon and Honey Blend:

Cinnamon is another ingredient known for its metabolism-boosting properties. Create a weight-loss elixir by mixing one tablespoon of honey with a teaspoon of cinnamon powder. Consume this blend with warm water, either in the morning or before bedtime. Cinnamon may help regulate blood sugar levels, reducing cravings and promoting a more stable energy balance throughout the day.

<u>Apple Cider Vinegar and Honey Tonic:</u>

Apple cider vinegar (ACV) is often associated with weight loss due to its potential to enhance feelings of fullness and improve metabolism. Create a powerful weight-loss tonic by combining one tablespoon of raw honey with two tablespoons of unfiltered apple cider vinegar in a glass of water. Drink this tonic before meals to potentially aid in digestion and support weight loss efforts.

<u>Directions</u>

Regardless of the honey weight-loss method chosen, it is crucial to incorporate these remedies into a comprehensive approach that includes a balanced diet and regular physical activity. Here are some general guidelines to maximize the effectiveness of honey for weight loss:

<u>Moderation is Key:</u>

While honey offers health benefits, it is essential to consume it in moderation. Excessive calorie intake, even from natural sources, can hinder weight loss efforts.

Choose Raw and Unprocessed:

Opt for raw, unprocessed honey to ensure you get the full spectrum of nutrients and enzymes that may contribute to weight loss.

Stay Hydrated:

Adequate hydration is crucial for overall health and can support weight loss. When consuming honey-infused drinks, ensure you also drink plenty of water throughout the day.

Combine With A Healthy Diet:

Honey should be seen as a complement to a balanced diet rich in fruits, vegetables, lean proteins, and whole grains. It is not a substitute for a healthy eating plan.

Regular Exercise:

Physical activity remains a cornerstone of any successful weight loss journey. Combine honey consumption with a consistent exercise routine to maximize results.

Natural Blood Purifier

A natural blood purifier is essential for eliminating toxins, promoting circulation, and supporting overall well-being. In this chapter, we explore a time-tested remedy using honey and other natural ingredients to cleanse and purify the blood.

Ingredients:

Raw Honey:

Raw, unfiltered honey is a key component of this natural blood purifier. Rich in antioxidants and enzymes, it helps eliminate harmful substances from the bloodstream.

Lemon Juice:

Packed with vitamin C, lemon juice supports liver function and aids in the detoxification process. Its acidic nature also helps balance pH levels in the body.

Turmeric:

Renowned for its anti-inflammatory properties, turmeric contains curcumin, a compound that enhances liver function and promotes the elimination of toxins.

Garlic:

Allicin, a potent compound found in garlic, has been shown to improve circulation and reduce the buildup of plaque in the arteries, contributing to a cleaner bloodstream.

Ginger:

Ginger possesses anti-inflammatory and antioxidant properties, promoting healthy blood flow and aiding in the removal of impurities.

<h1 style="text-align:center"><u>Directions:</u></h1>

To create this natural blood purifier, follow these simple steps:

1.) Combine two tablespoons of raw honey, the juice of one lemon, a teaspoon of turmeric powder, two crushed garlic cloves, and a tablespoon of grated ginger in a mixing bowl.

2.) Stir the ingredients thoroughly until a homogeneous mixture is formed.

3) Transfer the mixture to a glass jar with a lid, allowing it to sit for at least 12 hours to allow the flavors to meld.

4) Consume one tablespoon of the mixture daily, preferably in the morning on an empty stomach.

5) Continue this regimen for a minimum of two weeks to experience the full benefits of this natural blood purifier.

<u>Benefits:</u>

1) Detoxification: The combination of honey, lemon, turmeric, garlic, and ginger works synergistically to eliminate toxins from the bloodstream, promoting a natural and gentle detoxification process.

2) Improved Circulation: The ingredients in this remedy contribute to enhanced blood flow, reducing the risk of clot formation and promoting cardiovascular health.

3) Liver Support: The liver plays a crucial role in detoxification, and the components of this remedy support liver function, aiding in the breakdown and elimination of toxins.

4) Antioxidant Boost: The presence of antioxidants in raw honey, lemon, and turmeric helps combat free radicals, protecting cells from oxidative stress and contributing to overall health.

5) pH Balance: Lemon juice assists in maintaining a balanced pH level in the body, creating an environment less conducive to the proliferation of harmful microorganisms.

Conclusion

The book provides valuable insights, practical recipes, and herbal remedies that showcase the versatile nature of honey. With a focus on holistic approaches, this guide demonstrates how harnessing nature's sweet nectar can enhance various aspects of life, including health, skincare, and haircare.

Coution

any recipes or skincare rituals featured in this book should be tested on a small area of skin for potential allergies or adverse reactions before widespread application.